I0693270

M Joy
Reading

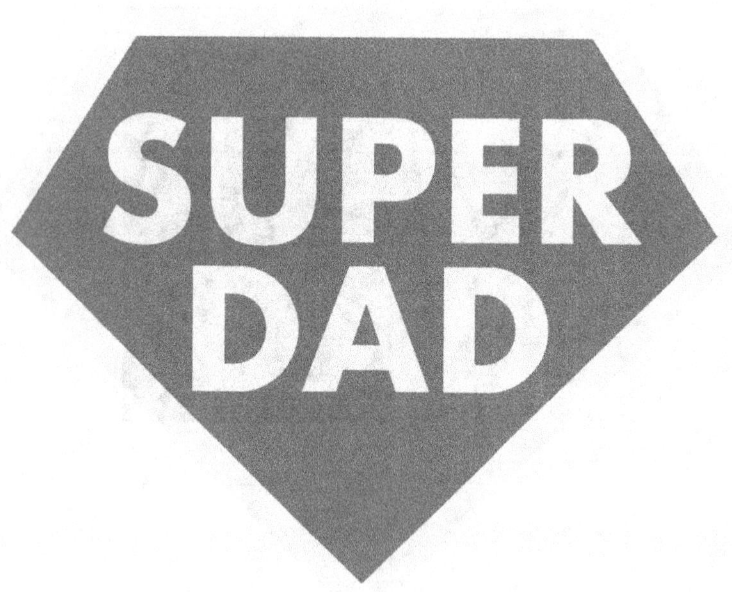
SUPER
DAD

BEST DAD EVER

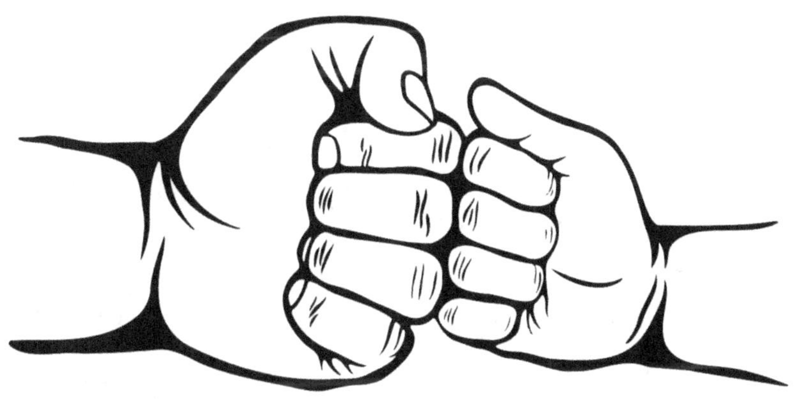

MARGARET ANN MCRAE

DAD JOKE

Looooooading....

please wait...

WHAT DID THE BUFFALO SAY TO HIS BABY BOY
WHEN PATERNITY LEAVE WAS OVER?

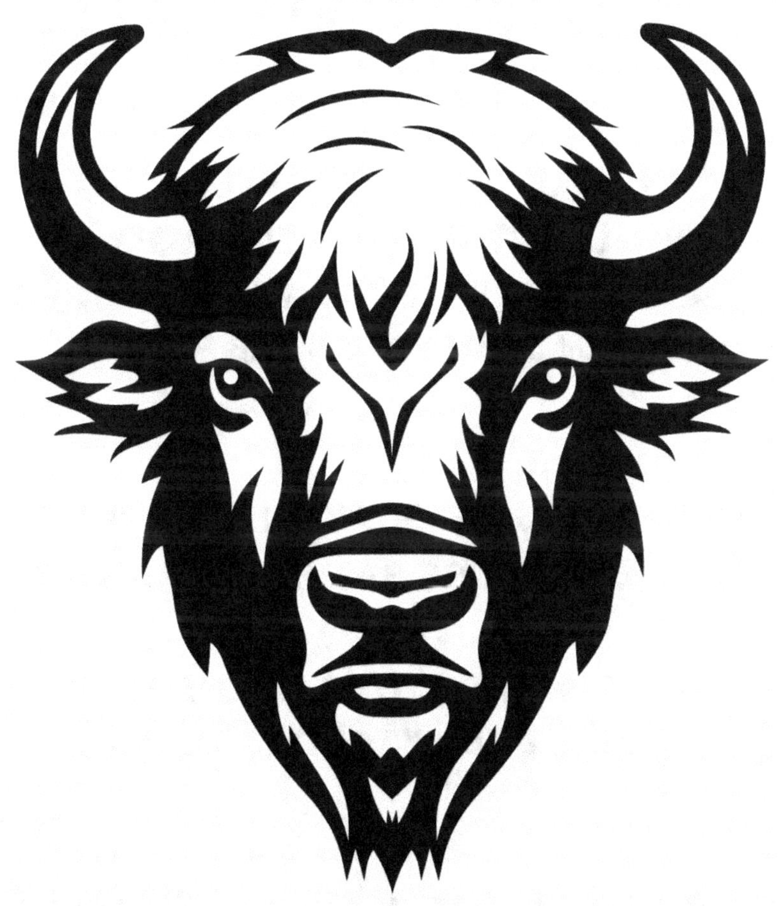

BISON!

Q: WHY DID THE NEW DAD BRING A LADDER TO THE HOSPITAL?
A: BECAUSE HE HEARD THE BABY WAS A LITTLE "UP" IN THE AIR.

Q: WHY DID THE NEW DAD CARRY A PENCIL TO THE DELIVERY ROOM?
A: IN CASE HE NEEDED TO DRAW SOME "DAD JOKES" ON THE BABY.

Q: DID YOU HEAR ABOUT THE NEW DAD WHO WORE SANDALS DURING LABOR?
A: HE WANTED TO BE PREPARED FOR THE "DAD-LY" DUTIES AHEAD.

Q: WHY WAS THE NEW DAD SO GOOD AT CHANGING DIAPERS?
A: HE HAD A "BRIEF" UNDERSTANDING OF THE SITUATION.

WHAT DO YOU CALL A NEWBORN BABY?

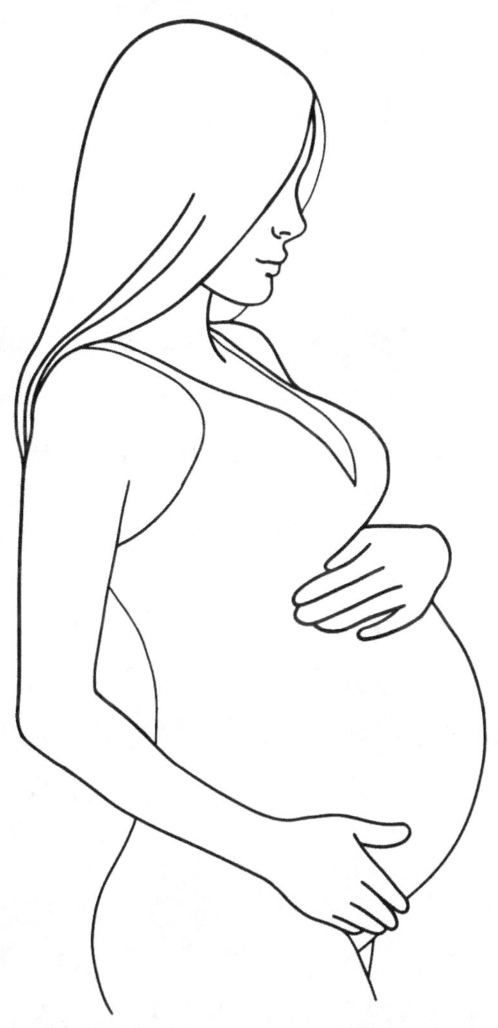

ANYTHING YOUR WIFE WANTS.

Q: WHY DID THE NEW DAD GET A JOB AT THE BAKERY?
A: BECAUSE HE KNEADED THE DOUGH FOR HIS NEW FAMILY.

Q: WHY DID THE NEW DAD GO TO THE BANK AFTER THE BABY WAS BORN?
A: TO OPEN A "SAVINGS" ACCOUNT FOR FUTURE DIAPER EXPENSES.

Q: WHY DID THE NEW DAD TAKE UP GARDENING?
A: HE WANTED TO UNDERSTAND THE "ROOTS" OF PARENTHOOD.

Q: WHY DID THE NEW DAD START TALKING TO THE WALLS?
A: HE HEARD IT WAS THE FIRST SIGN OF BECOMING A "DAD JOKE" EXPERT

Q: WHY DID THE BABY CRAWL ACROSS THE STREET?

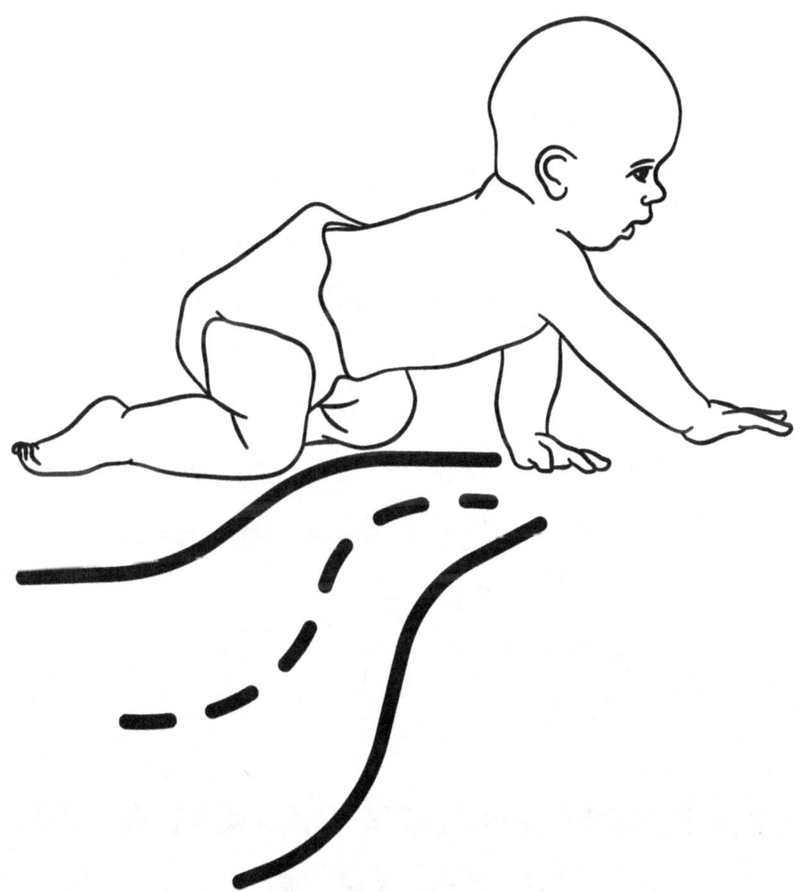

A: HE SAW THE ONE OBJECT YOU TOLD HIM HE COULDN'T PLAY WITH.

Q: WHY WAS THE NEW DAD ALWAYS
A HIT AT PARTIES?
A: BECAUSE HE KNEW HOW TO "DAD
DANCE" LIKE A PRO.

Q: WHY DID THE NEW DAD PUT A
CLOCK IN HIS BABY'S ROOM?
A: TO "TOCK" ABOUT THE PRECIOUS
MOMENTS WITH HIS LITTLE ONE.

Q: WHY DID THE NEW DAD KEEP A
HAMMER IN HIS DIAPER BAG?
A: FOR "EMERGENCY REPAIRS"
DURING PLAYDATES.

Q: WHY DID THE NEW DAD GET A JOB
AT THE ZOO?
A: BECAUSE HE WANTED TO WORK
WITH "LITTLE MONKEYS" LIKE HIS
OWN.

Q: WHAT DO YOU CALL A BABY POTATO?

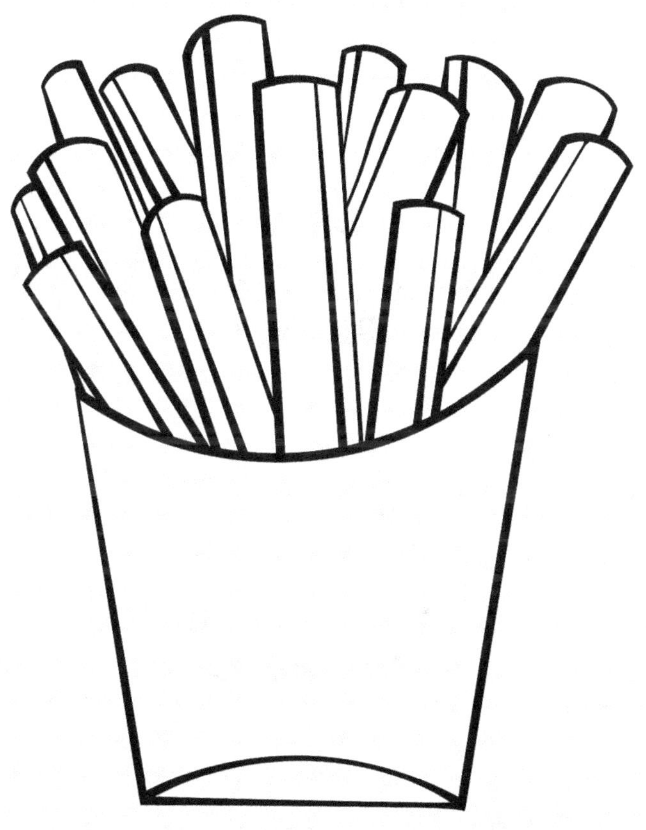

A: A SMALL FRY.

Q: WHY DID THE NEW DAD BRING A CAMERA TO THE CHANGING TABLE?
A: TO CAPTURE THE "UNFORGETTABLE" MOMENTS OF DIAPER DUTY.

Q: WHY DID THE NEW DAD BECOME A CHEF?
A: TO MASTER THE ART OF "BABY FOOD" CUISINE.

Q: WHY DID THE NEW DAD CARRY A MAP EVERYWHERE?
A: TO NAVIGATE THE "TERRITORY" OF FATHERHOOD.

Q: WHY DID THE NEW DAD JOIN A SUPPORT GROUP FOR SLEEP-DEPRIVED PARENTS?
A: HE NEEDED A PLACE TO SHARE HIS "TIRED" JOKES.

WHAT DO YOU CALL A COW THAT HAD A BABY?

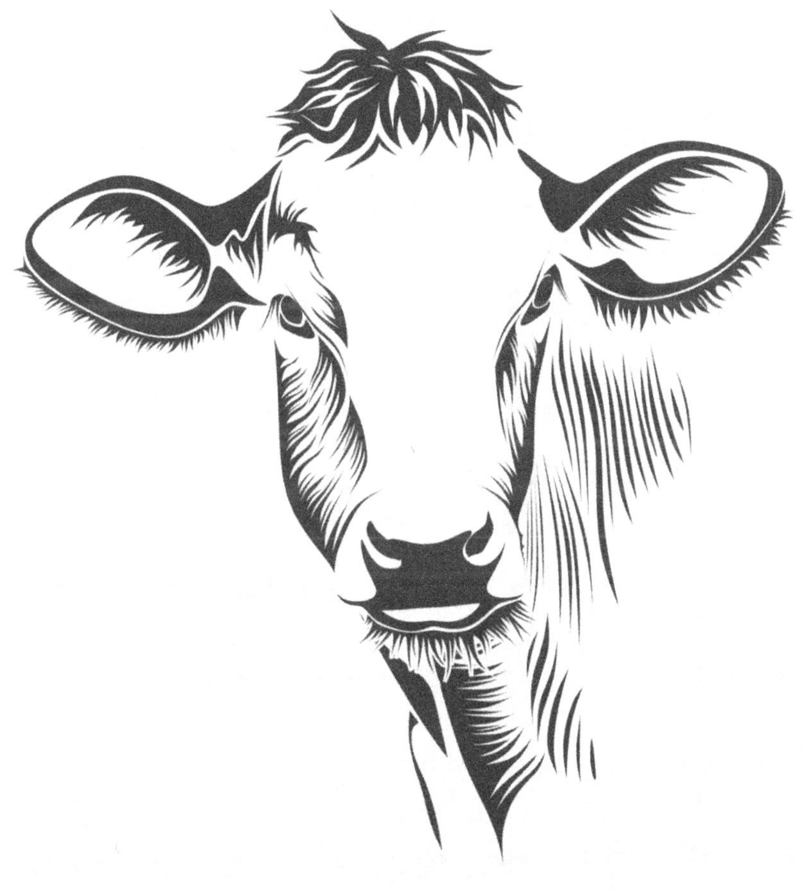

DE-CALF-INATED.

Q: WHY DID THE NEW DAD BUY STOCK IN BABY FORMULA COMPANIES?
A: HE BELIEVED IN INVESTING IN HIS BABY'S "FUTURE GROWTH."

Q: WHY DID THE NEW DAD START STUDYING ASTRONOMY?
A: HE WANTED TO UNDERSTAND THE "CONSTELLATIONS" OF PARENTHOOD.

Q: WHY DID THE NEW DAD TAKE UP PAINTING?
A: TO CAPTURE THE COLORFUL CHAOS OF FATHERHOOD ON CANVAS.

Q: WHY DID THE NEW DAD BECOME A BARBER?
A: TO MASTER THE ART OF "TODDLER HAIRCUTS."

Q: WHEN DO PARENTS CHANGE THE MOST BABY DIAPERS?

A: IN THE WEE WEE HOURS.

Q: WHY DID THE NEW DAD BUY A SUPERHERO COSTUME?
A: TO BECOME HIS BABY'S "SUPER-DAD" IN TIMES OF NEED.

Q: WHY DID THE NEW DAD BRING A SNORKEL TO BATH TIME?
A: HE HEARD IT WAS THE BEST WAY TO "DIVE" INTO FATHERHOOD.

Q: WHY DID THE NEW DAD START COLLECTING RUBBER DUCKS?
A: FOR HIS BABY'S "QUACK" ADDICTION.

Q: WHY DID THE NEW DAD BRING A RULER TO THE HOSPITAL?
A: BECAUSE HE WANTED TO MEASURE UP TO THE CHALLENGE OF FATHERHOOD.

Q: DO YOU KNOW WHY BABIES BORN ON HOLIDAYS ARE MORE THAN LIKELY TO BE LITTLE GIRLS?

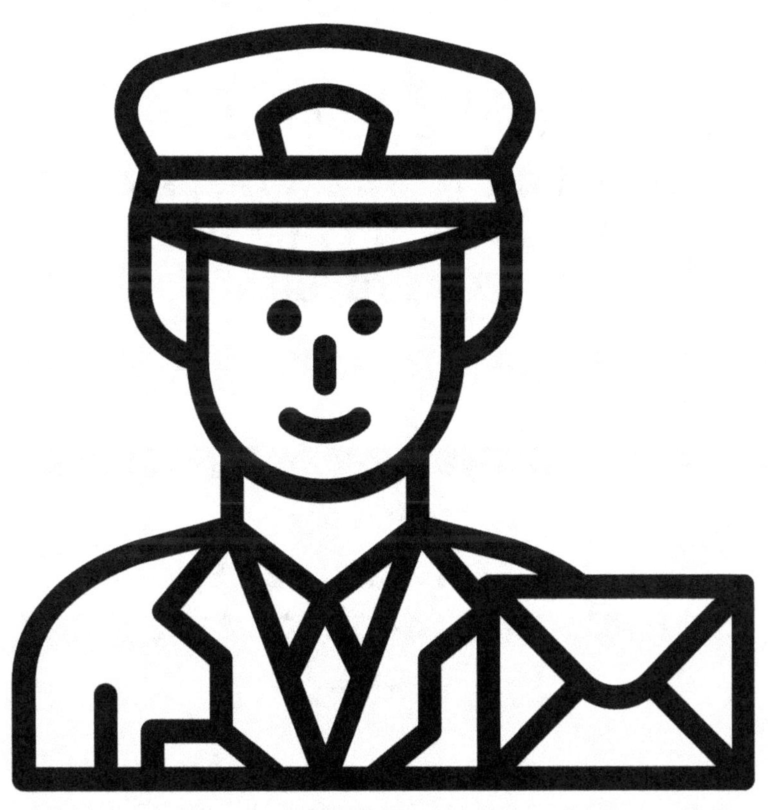

A: BECAUSE THERE IS NO MAIL DELIVERY ON HOLIDAYS.

Q: WHY DID THE NEW DAD START PRACTICING MAGIC TRICKS?
A: TO MASTER THE ART OF MAKING TANTRUMS DISAPPEAR.

Q: WHY DID THE NEW DAD BRING A TOOLBOX TO THE NURSERY?
A: TO FIX ANYTHING THAT NEEDED A "DAD'S TOUCH."

Q: WHY DID THE NEW DAD BECOME A COMEDIAN?
A: BECAUSE HE ALREADY HAD AN AUDIENCE THAT LAUGHED AT HIS EVERY MOVE.

Q: WHY DID THE NEW DAD START LEARNING ORIGAMI?
A: TO FOLD HIS WAY OUT OF TRICKY PARENTING SITUATIONS.

WHAT DO BABIES USUALLY PLAY IN A BAND?

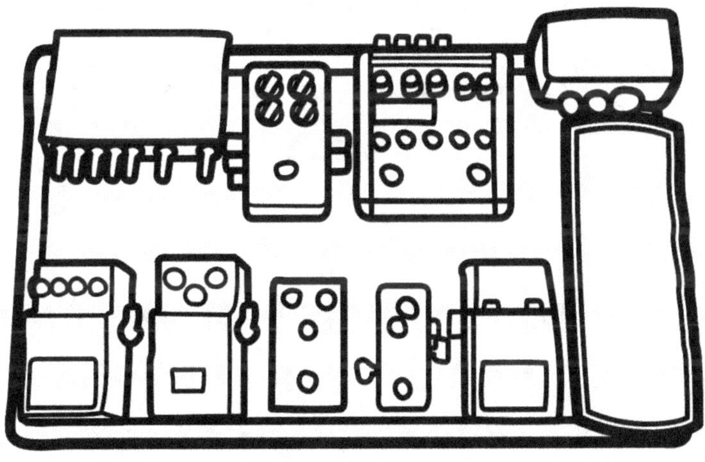

A: THEY PLAY GUITARS HOOKED UP TO 'WAAH!
WAAH! PEDALS'.

Q: WHY DID THE NEW DAD START A BAND WITH OTHER DADS?
A: BECAUSE THEY WANTED TO ROCK THE BABY TO SLEEP WITH LULLABIES.

Q: WHY DID THE NEW DAD ENROLL IN A YOGA CLASS?
A: TO MASTER THE ART OF "PARENTAL BALANCE."

Q: WHY DID THE NEW DAD INVEST IN NOISE-CANCELING HEADPHONES?
A: TO TUNE OUT THE CHAOS AND ENJOY A MOMENT OF PEACE.

Q: WHY DID THE NEW DAD START TELLING BABY-THEMED PUNS?
A: BECAUSE HE WANTED TO "RATTLE" OFF SOME JOKES.

**DO YOU KNOW WHAT A BABY COMPUTER CALLS
HIS OLD MAN?**

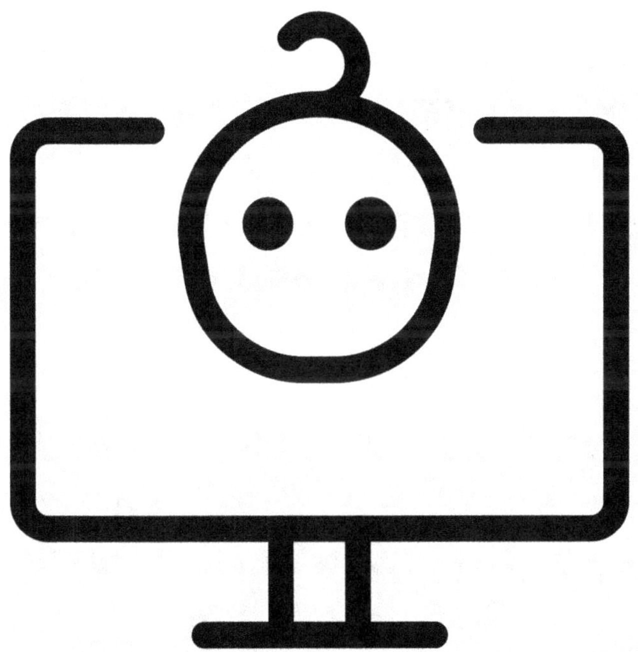

DATA.

Q: WHY DID THE NEW DAD BECOME A STORYTELLER?
A: TO WEAVE TALES OF ADVENTURE FOR HIS LITTLE ONE.

Q: WHY DID THE NEW DAD BUY A MINI BASKETBALL HOOP FOR THE NURSERY?
A: TO START TRAINING HIS BABY FOR FUTURE CHAMPIONSHIPS.

Q: WHY DID THE NEW DAD START PRACTICING BEATBOXING?
A: TO ENTERTAIN HIS BABY WITH RHYTHMIC SOUNDS.

Q: WHY DID THE NEW DAD BECOME A DIY EXPERT?
A: TO BUILD MEMORIES WHILE BUILDING FURNITURE FOR THE NURSERY.

DID YOU HEAR WHAT THE COUPLE WHO MET WHILE WORKING AT AN INSTRUCTION BOOK COMPANY NAMED THEIR KID?

MANUEL.

Q: WHY DID THE NEW DAD START TAKING COOKING CLASSES?
A: TO WHIP UP DELICIOUS MEALS FOR HIS GROWING FAMILY.

Q: WHY DID THE NEW DAD START WATCHING CHILDREN'S CARTOONS?
A: TO STAY UPDATED ON THE LATEST TRENDS IN KIDS' ENTERTAINMENT.

Q: WHY DID THE NEW DAD BRING A PILLOW TO THE DELIVERY ROOM?
A: TO CATCH UP ON SOME MUCH-NEEDED SLEEP DURING LABOR.

Q: WHY DID THE NEW DAD BECOME A CROSSWORD ENTHUSIAST?
A: TO SHARPEN HIS WIT AND SOLVE PARENTING PUZZLES.

WHAT DID THE FIRE SAY TO HER HUSBAND AFTER THEIR SON'S BIRTH?

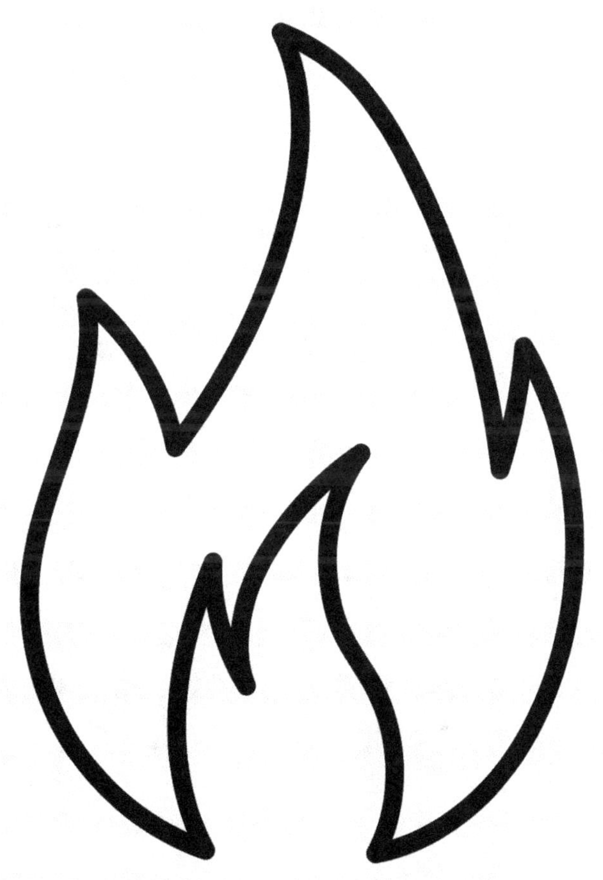

A: "HONEY... THIS IS ARSON."

Q: WHY DID THE NEW DAD START PRACTICING HIS VENTRILOQUISM SKILLS?
A: TO ENTERTAIN HIS BABY WITH "TALKING" TOYS.

Q: WHY DID THE NEW DAD INVEST IN A BABY CARRIER WITH POCKETS?
A: TO STORE SNACKS FOR HIMSELF DURING LONG WALKS WITH THE BABY.

Q: WHY DID THE NEW DAD START LEARNING SIGN LANGUAGE?
A: TO COMMUNICATE WITH HIS BABY BEFORE THEY COULD SPEAK.

Q: WHY DID THE NEW DAD BRING A CAMERA CREW TO THE HOSPITAL?
A: TO CAPTURE THE "BLOCKBUSTER" MOMENT OF BECOMING A DAD.

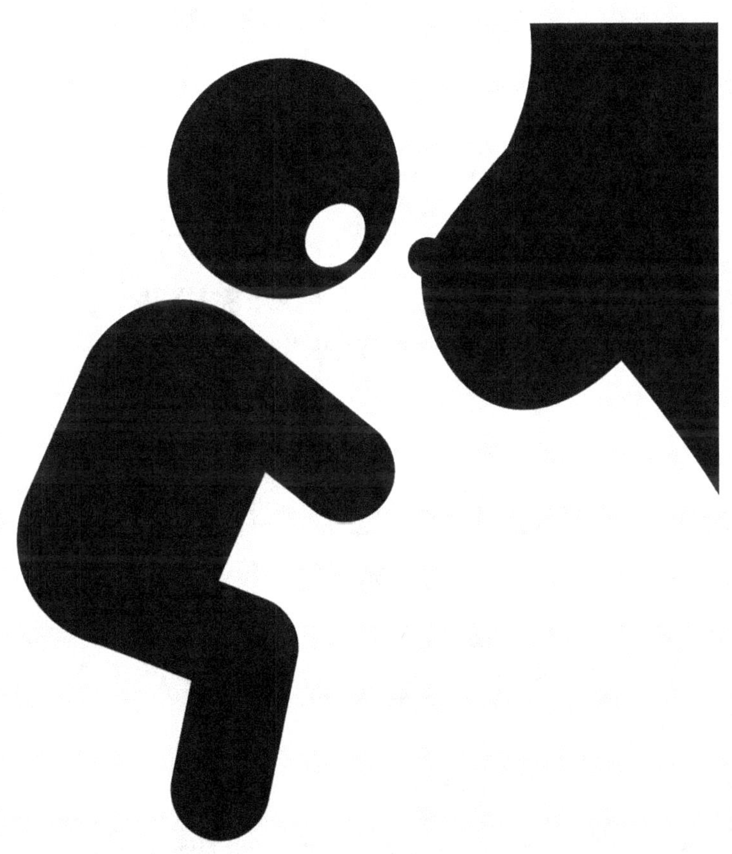

"I DON'T ALWAYS DRINK MILK. BUT WHEN I DO, I PREFER DOS TETAS."

– THE MOST INTERESTING BABY IN THE WORLD.

Q: WHY DID THE NEW DAD START TAKING BALLET LESSONS?
A: TO PERFECT HIS "DAD DANCE" MOVES WITH GRACE AND ELEGANCE.

Q: WHY DID THE NEW DAD START COLLECTING COMIC BOOKS?
A: TO SHARE HIS LOVE FOR SUPERHEROES WITH HIS LITTLE SIDEKICK.

Q: WHY DID THE NEW DAD BECOME A POET?
A: TO PEN HEARTFELT VERSES DEDICATED TO HIS BUNDLE OF JOY.

Q: WHY DID THE NEW DAD START WATCHING COOKING SHOWS?
A: TO MASTER THE ART OF PREPARING BABY-FRIENDLY MEALS.

Q: WHY IS THAT BABY STILL IN DIAPERS?

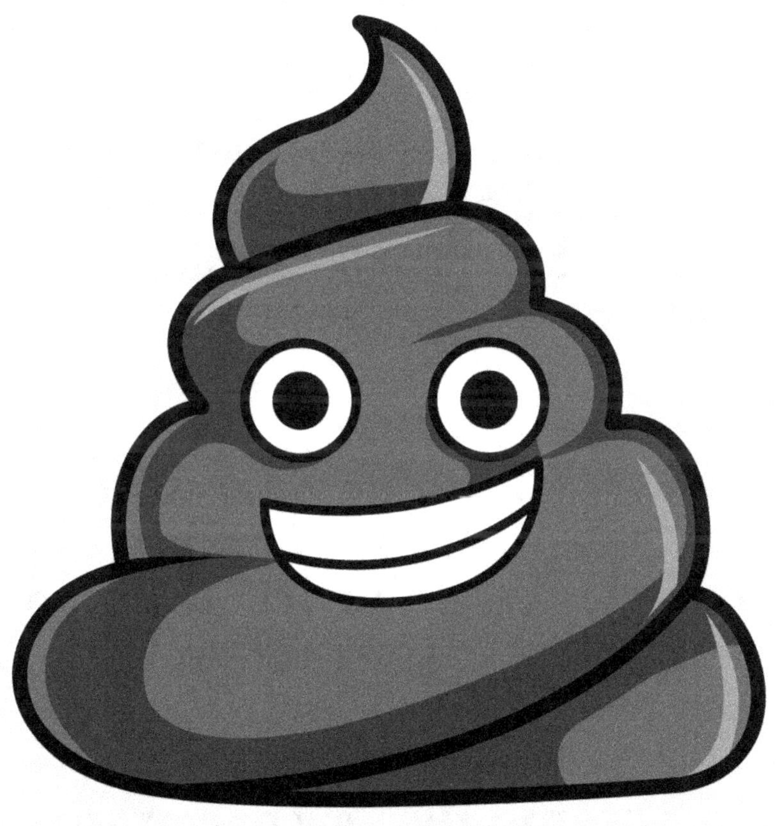

A: I'LL GIVE YOU TWO REASONS: NUMBER 1 AND
NUMBER 2.

Q: WHY DID THE NEW DAD BRING A COMPASS TO THE DELIVERY ROOM?
A: TO NAVIGATE THE JOURNEY OF FATHERHOOD WITH PRECISION.

Q: WHY DID THE NEW DAD START PRACTICING BEATBOXING?
A: TO CREATE FUNKY BEATS FOR IMPROMPTU BABY DANCE PARTIES.

Q: WHY DID THE NEW DAD JOIN A PARENTING BOOK CLUB?
A: TO EXCHANGE "DADVICE" AND BOND WITH FELLOW FATHERS.

Q: WHY DID THE NEW DAD START COLLECTING ACTION FIGURES?
A: TO INTRODUCE HIS BABY TO THE WORLD OF SUPERHEROES AND VILLAINS.

MY NEWBORN SON MADE SUCH A FUSS WHEN THE
DOCTOR CUT HIS UMBILICAL CORD.

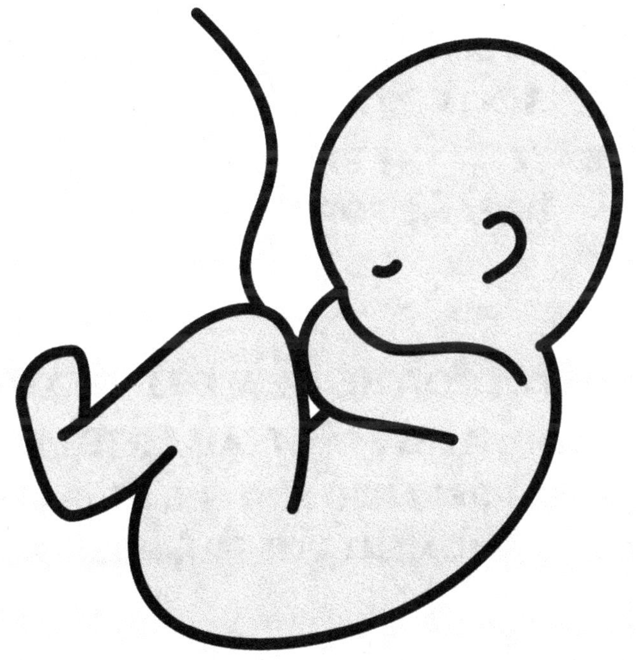

HE HAD REALLY GROWN ATTACHED TO IT.

Q: WHY DID THE NEW DAD BECOME A PUPPETEER?

A: TO PUT ON ENTERTAINING SHOWS FOR HIS LITTLE AUDIENCE.

Q: WHY DID THE NEW DAD BRING A TELESCOPE TO THE NURSERY?

A: TO GAZE AT THE STARS AND DREAM BIG DREAMS FOR HIS CHILD.

Q: WHY DID THE NEW DAD START LEARNING MARTIAL ARTS?

A: TO BE PREPARED FOR THE "KARATE-CHOP" MOMENTS OF PARENTING.

Q: WHY DID THE NEW DAD START GARDENING?

A: TO TEACH HIS CHILD THE BEAUTY OF NURTURING AND GROWTH.

WHAT DO YOU DO WHEN YOUR BABY IS BEING FUSSY?

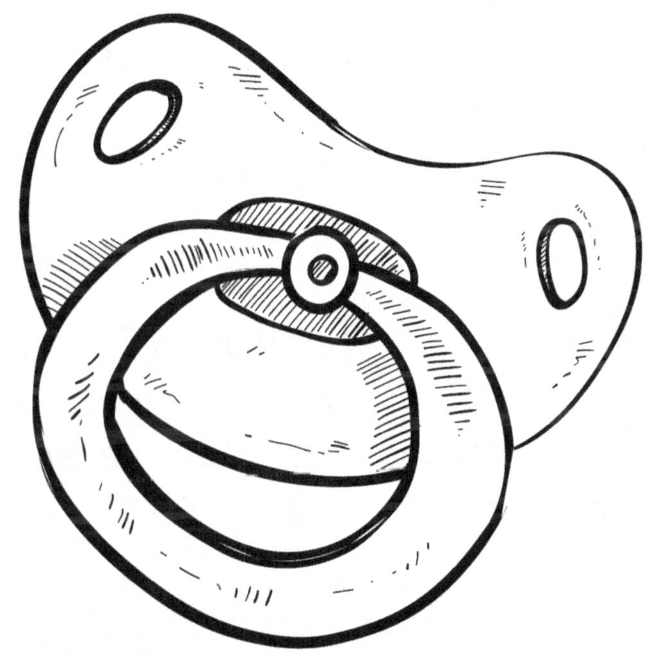

I'LL PACIFY IT.

Q: WHY DID THE NEW DAD BUY A CLOWN COSTUME?

A: TO BE THE LIFE OF THE PARTY AT HIS BABY'S BIRTHDAY CELEBRATIONS.

Q: WHY DID THE NEW DAD START LEARNING MAGIC TRICKS?

A: TO DAZZLE HIS BABY WITH ILLUSIONS AND WONDER.

Q: WHY DID THE NEW DAD BECOME A CROSSWORD PUZZLE ENTHUSIAST?

A: TO EXERCISE HIS BRAIN WHILE WAITING FOR THE BABY TO SLEEP.

Q: WHY DID THE NEW DAD BRING A DICTIONARY TO THE DELIVERY ROOM?

A: TO FIND THE PERFECT WORDS TO DESCRIBE THE OVERWHELMING JOY OF FATHERHOOD.

WHY DIDN'T THE BABY WANT TO BE BORN?

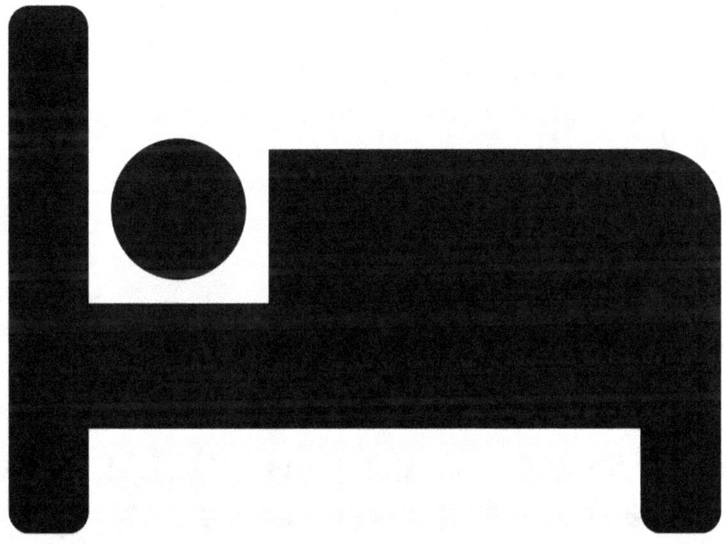

A: BECAUSE IT DIDN'T WANT TO GIVE UP ITS FREE
WOMB AND BOARD!

Q: WHY DID THE NEW DAD START LEARNING HOW TO PLAY MUSICAL INSTRUMENTS?
A: TO SERENADE HIS BABY WITH SWEET MELODIES AND LULLABIES.

Q: WHY DID THE NEW DAD JOIN A BABY SWIM CLASS?
A: TO MAKE A SPLASH AND BOND WITH HIS LITTLE ONE IN THE WATER.

Q: WHY DID THE NEW DAD START COLLECTING BOARD GAMES?
A: TO ENJOY FAMILY GAME NIGHTS AND CREATE LASTING MEMORIES WITH HIS CHILD.

Q: WHY DID THE NEW DAD BRING A GUITAR TO THE HOSPITAL?
A: TO STRUM SOME SOOTHING TUNES FOR THE NEWBORN.

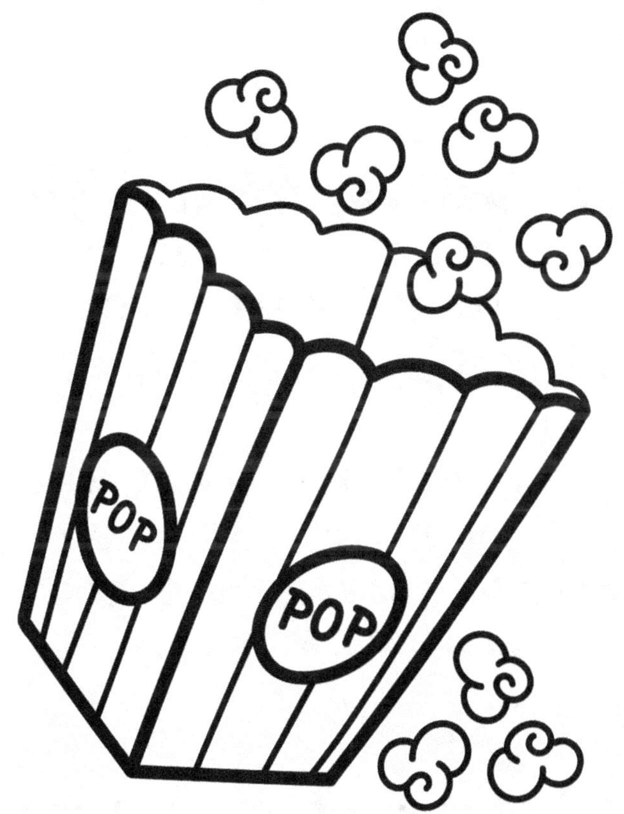

A: "WHERE IS POP CORN?"

Q: WHY DID THE NEW DAD START LEARNING HOW TO JUGGLE?
A: TO MASTER THE ART OF MULTITASKING AS A PARENT.

Q: WHY DID THE NEW DAD BRING A MINI TRAMPOLINE TO THE NURSERY?
A: TO BOUNCE BACK FROM THE CHALLENGES OF PARENTHOOD.

Q: WHY DID THE NEW DAD START LEARNING HOW TO KNIT?
A: TO CRAFT ADORABLE BABY BOOTIES AND HATS WITH LOVE.

Q: WHY DID THE NEW DAD BECOME A BIRDWATCHER?
A: TO TEACH HIS CHILD ABOUT THE WONDERS OF NATURE.

Q: WHERE DO BABY CATS LEARN TO SWIM?

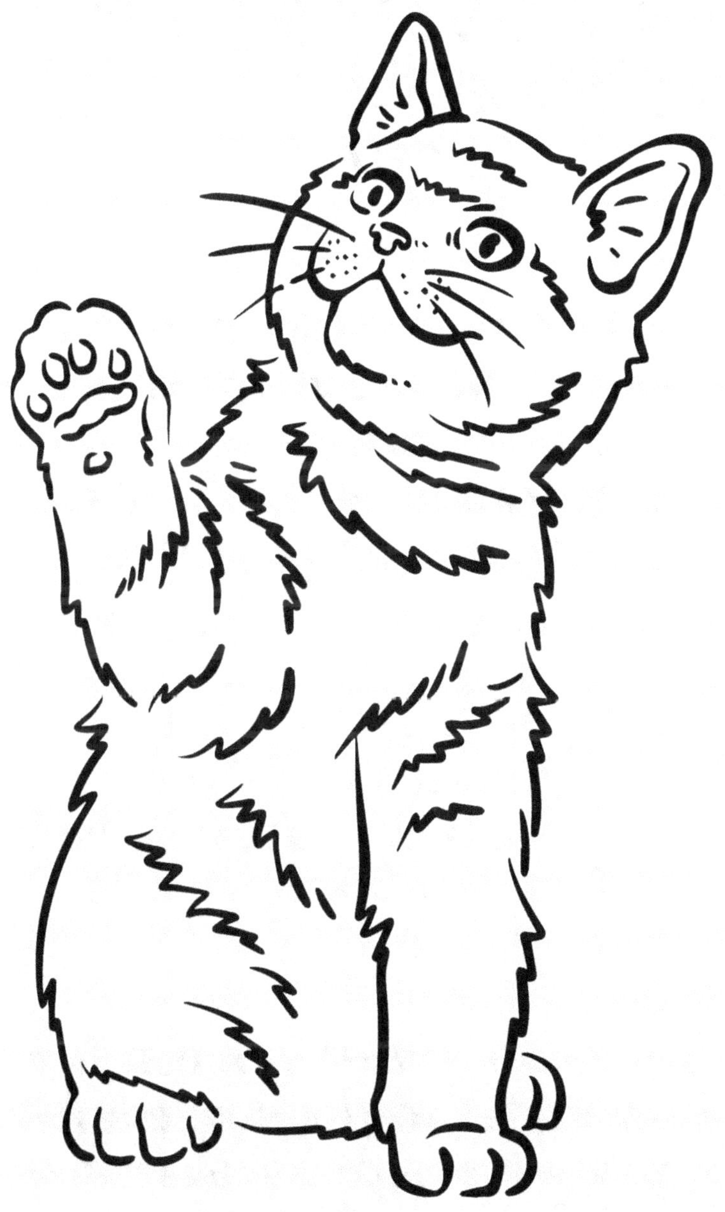

A: THE KITTY POOL.

Q: WHY DID THE NEW DAD BRING A MAP TO THE DELIVERY ROOM?
A: TO NAVIGATE THE TWISTS AND TURNS OF LABOR.

Q: WHY DID THE NEW DAD START PRACTICING HIS VENTRILOQUISM SKILLS?
A: TO ENTERTAIN THE BABY WITH FUNNY VOICES AND CHARACTERS.

Q: WHY DID THE NEW DAD BECOME A CONNOISSEUR OF BABY FOOD?
A: TO DEVELOP A PALATE FOR PUREED PEAS AND MASHED BANANAS.

Q: WHY DID THE NEW DAD BRING A WHISTLE TO THE NURSERY?
A: TO REFEREE SIBLING SQUABBLES AND MAINTAIN ORDER.

Q: WHAT DO YOU GIVE A PIG WITH A DIAPER RASH?

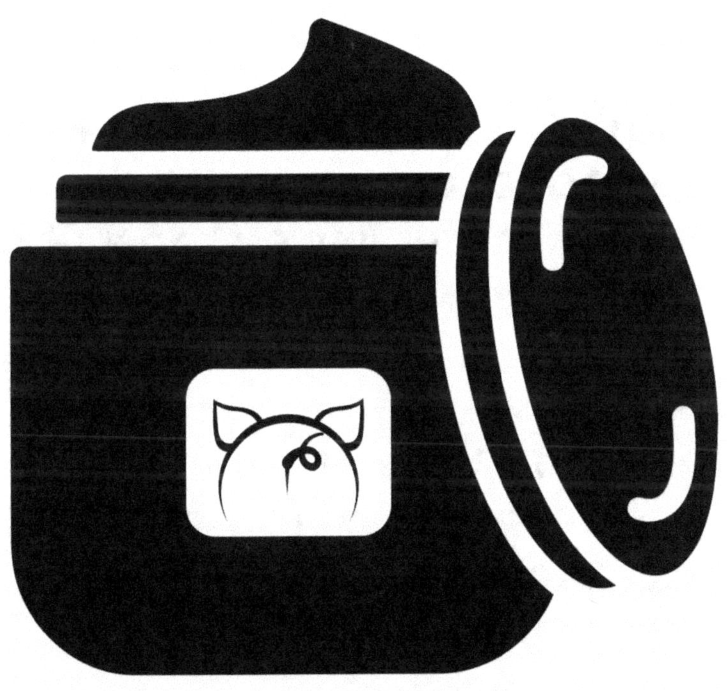

A: OINKMENT.

Q: WHY DID THE NEW DAD START LEARNING HOW TO MAKE BALLOON ANIMALS?
A: TO AMAZE HIS CHILD WITH WHIMSICAL CREATIONS AT BIRTHDAY PARTIES.

Q: WHY DID THE NEW DAD BRING A TELESCOPE TO BEDTIME STORIES?
A: TO EXPLORE THE UNIVERSE TOGETHER THROUGH THE PAGES OF A BOOK.

Q: WHY DID THE NEW DAD START LEARNING ORIGAMI?
A: TO FOLD PAPER CRANES AND TEACH HIS CHILD THE ART OF PATIENCE.

Q: WHY DID THE NEW DAD BECOME A STORYTELLER?
A: TO SPIN TALES OF ADVENTURE AND WONDER FOR HIS LITTLE ONE.

WHAT'S A GROUP OF CHUBBY NEWBORNS
CALLED?

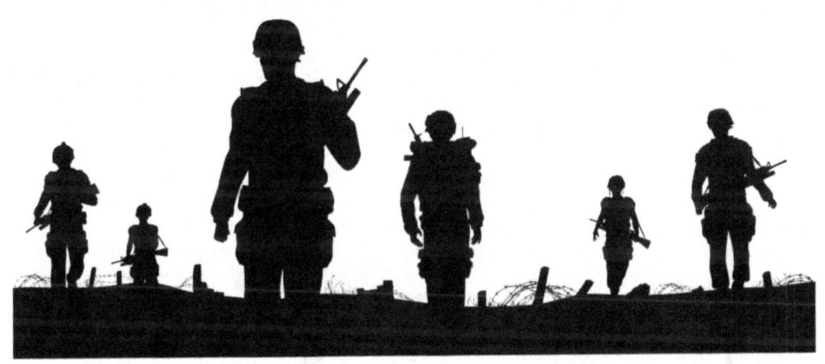

A: HEAVY INFANTRY

Q: WHY DID THE NEW DAD BRING A HARMONICA TO THE NURSERY?
A: TO PLAY SWEET MELODIES AND LULLABIES FOR THE BABY.

Q: WHY DID THE NEW DAD START COLLECTING STAMPS?
A: TO PASS DOWN A HOBBY AND CREATE A FAMILY TRADITION.

Q: WHY DID THE NEW DAD JOIN A BABY SIGN LANGUAGE CLASS?
A: TO COMMUNICATE WITH HIS CHILD BEFORE THEY COULD SPEAK.

Q: WHY DID THE NEW DAD START LEARNING MAGIC TRICKS?
A: TO PERFORM FEATS OF ILLUSION AND WONDER FOR THE BABY.

WHAT WOULD YOU CALL A BABY WHO'S A STAND-UP COMEDIAN?

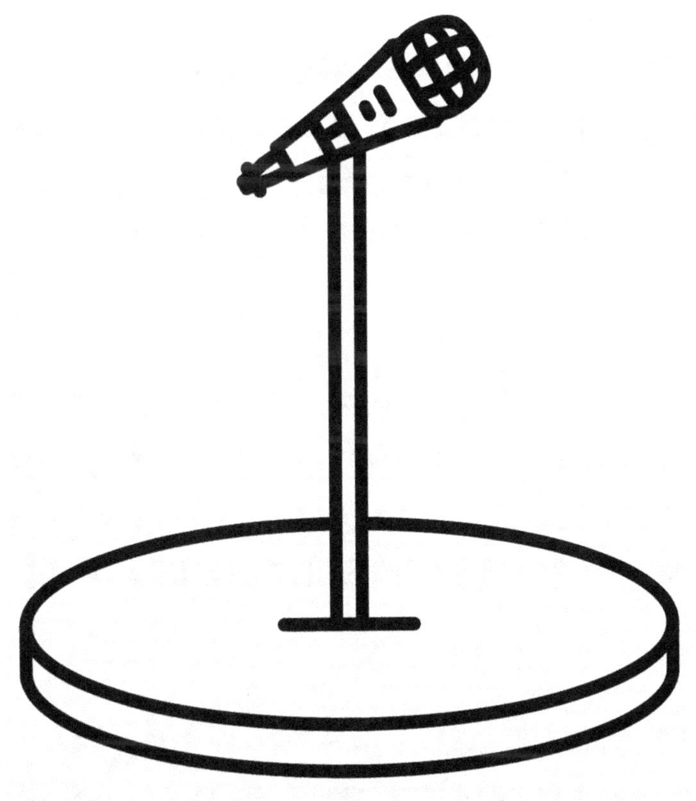

A: A KIDDER.

Q: WHY DID THE NEW DAD BRING A TELESCOPE TO THE PARK?
A: TO STARGAZE AND DREAM BIG DREAMS WITH HIS CHILD.

Q: WHY DID THE NEW DAD START LEARNING HOW TO MAKE POTTERY?
A: TO CRAFT PERSONALIZED KEEPSAKES AND GIFTS FOR THE FAMILY.

Q: WHY DID THE NEW DAD BECOME A COLLECTOR OF CHILDREN'S BOOKS?
A: TO BUILD A LIBRARY OF STORIES AND ADVENTURES FOR BEDTIME READING.

Q: WHAT DID MASTER YODA SAY WHEN LUKE SLICED THE BALL ONTO THE NEXT FAIRWAY OVER?
A: "MAY THE 'FORES' BE WITH YOU…"

I SAW A BABY OWL CAUGHT IN THE RAIN.

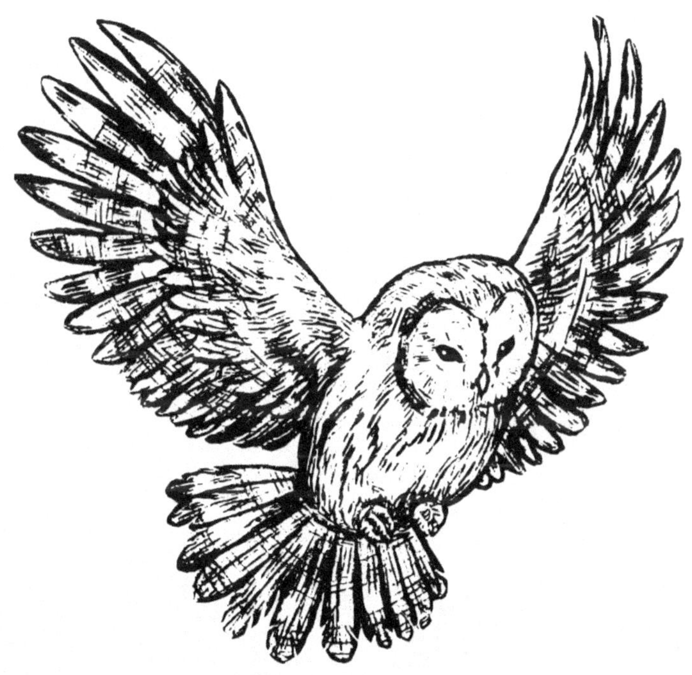

IT WAS A MOIST OWLET.